MW01109899

Warning-Disclaimer
The purpose of this book is to educate and inspire. It is not intended to treat, cure or diagnose any disease, nor take the place of working with a qualified natural health practitioner or other health care provider.

About The Author:

LeAnn has quickly become the leading authority on "putting it all together" so individuals and organizations have the ability to have incredible energy, amazing productivity and an overall healthy life. After getting a degree in exercise science and becoming a certified personal trainer for 7 years LeAnn learned quickly that being healthy was not just about exercise. This moved her to get a naturopathic degree and then from there a masters degree in Live Vegan Nutrition. She became aware that being completely healthy was more than just food as well. She learned it was the ability to balance what goes into your mind, your body and the habits that form your lifestyle. She is the author of the bestselling book "Get Healthy Now," runs a highly successful consulting practice and is a sought after speaker. Her mission is to see people realize how good they can feel when they are given the proper tools and information.

Help others to Get Healthy NOW by sharing this book with your group or organization.

Get Healthy NOW...3 Simple Steps to boundless energy, incredible productivity and the most amazing YOU.

The tips and strategies shared in this book will change your entire future. They will impact every area of your life. Apply even a few of these simple and practical steps and you will start to see the cumulative effects of positive change over time. Read and share these steps daily for best results. All of this life changing information is only $19.95!

Special Quantity Discounts:

5-20 Books	$17.95 each
21-99 Books	$16.95 each
100-499 Books	$13.95 each
500-999 Books	$9.95 each
1000+ Books	$6.95 each

To place an order contact LeAnn at:
269.204.6525 or Frontdesk@NewHopeHealth.com

"LeAnn Fritz is amazing! **Get Healthy Now!** *is packed with valuable information. It helped me reduce my stress, sleep better, make better eating choices, and remember to make my health a priority. It's so easy to forget about health if you're working too much. I followed her program and have never felt better. Times have changed and it's more important than ever to learn what LeAnn teaches and follow through with it. I highly recommend LeAnn's program whether it's for you, your company, friends or family and think every company should offer it to their employees!"*

– Diane Polnow, Director of Business Development, American Express

Table of Contents

Introduction

You are in the right place. Finally, you will get real answers and practical steps on how to increase your energy, have explosive productivity and be the most amazing you!

Being healthy is about more than just food. It's a mind-set. It's about thinking differently which will enable you to LIVE differently. Although physical nutrition is important, it is also essential that you put great nutrition in to your mind and powerful habits into your life. That's what makes this book different from other health books that you may have read. You were engineered to be healthy in every way, NOW!

Getting healthy NOW is both a journey and a point in time. While it can take some time to reach your long term health goals, getting healthy NOW starts NOW, with a decision to TAKE ACTION and start receiving the fruits of those decisions! You will gain the mindset and nutritional insight you need to get healthy and stay healthy! It's not about a quick fix or another diet...it's about making lifestyle habits that become easier and easier over time.

Congratulations on your choice to take the first step NOW by reading this book. This book is divided into three sections. The first section is about fixing your mind and thinking. If you think right about getting Healthy NOW, you will be empowered to make changes faster and with more ease. The second section discusses tips that will impact you physically with food and nutrition. Many of these steps are SO simple you will be able to apply them instantly. This is not a diet mentality. Diets are restrictive and don't work. There is no hope in following a diet. A lifestyle change over time however is both sustainable and enjoyable. The final section of the book deals with lifestyle habits. This section will teach you some incredible tips that will have a tide of positive effects that will infiltrate all areas of your work, family and personal life.

If you love to read, just dive in. If you're not a big reader this book will still work for you too. Just read a tip each morning and a tip each night. This will only take about 5 minutes per day. Choosing to fill out the Get Healthy NOW action steps that go with each tip will cause you to progress even faster! If you don't know what to write, take a break and come back to it. The tips are incredible tools to help you succeed but they are activated when you personalize them by answering the questions. The questions are designed to empower you to APPLY each concept. So here's to you Getting Healthy NOW! Mark my words...TODAY is a day to remember. You will never be the same!

Section 1 – What You Put in Your Mind

What you put in your MIND will either increase or poison your energy, productivity and your ability to achieve the best version of YOU possible. If you put good, intellectual, positive things in, you will act accordingly and build great habits. In contrast, if you focus and fill your mind with negative or harmful thoughts, you will manifest poor habits. Let's get healthy NOW by changing the way we think and fuel our minds!

I am Responsible

Taking responsibility for what is currently happening in your life is the first step toward having hope and gaining control. If you see yourself as a victim, you have given the control of your life away. The truth is that in most cases, we earn our health, finances, and relationships. If you continually spend more money than you earn, you will continually live in fear of not having enough. Your mind will never be clear and your focus will constantly be on just "getting by". This cycle works both ways. If you consistently make wise investments and spend money reasonably, you will eventually have excess/ abundance that allows you to meet your needs with ease and give to others.

These principles apply to every area of life. If for example, you are always late, sometimes it's easy to feel like that's just "how you are", but there is hope. If you look at your habits there are likely several logical reasons why you are late. After careful analysis you will see that the things which make you late are nearly all choices that you make. NOW it is within your power to make other choices that will let you be on time. It's easy to blame your kids, spouse, weather, traffic and many other things, but that will still leave you feeling stuck! Think about what would happen if you got up earlier, more accurately estimated the time it takes for you to get ready, leave extra time for traffic, or do things the night before to prepare. These are a few examples of areas in which people tend to blame external circumstances for internal problems.

While we are not always responsible for what happens to us, we most definitely are responsible for how we respond to what happens to us. When you relinquish personal responsibility (blame external conditions) you forfeit your ability to change.

- List at least one circumstance in your life that you are blame-shifting or making excuses for. What is really going on? What are the obstacles that make this issue challenging? List at least 3 SPECIFIC steps that you could take to turn this around.

_____

_____

_____

_____

_____

_____

_____

_____

_____

_____

_____

_____

"No one can do your push-ups for you."

- Jim Rohn

Your Thoughts Change Your Life

The things that we do, both good and bad, all start in the mind. Those thoughts eventually become actions, habits and behaviors. What we think about is critical to having optimal energy, productivity, and overall balance in life.

Our thoughts are constant conversations with ourselves. Too often they are automatic and we are totally disengaged in the conversation, just allowing them to happen. It can be helpful to have a specific mantra, quote, or verse to come back to when your thoughts go in a direction that is not helpful. Here is a filter to work through: Seek to only allow yourself to think on things that are true.

We have all had times where we allow ourselves to dwell on or worry about assumptions or perceptions that aren't even real, positive, productive, or up-lifting. You can take control of your thoughts NOW. It helps to understand how the brain works. The goal here is to have a realistic grip on reality. For example, let's say that your job feels overwhelming with all the things that you have to do. Your mind may automatically run to thoughts like, "I will never get it all done". These thoughts are unproductive, even if they are accurate (which they usually aren't). If you tell your brain that you won't get it done, your brain will seek to produce that result. However, if you replace that thought with a more productive thought, such as "I can only do one thing at a time", or "How can I get more done in less time?", your brain will start working on the answer to this question. You may then realize that there is something you can delegate, or a task that is higher priority that will allow other items to take care of themselves. You may even find that the most important thing you can do is to go outside and take a 10 minute break so you can restore your energy and get balanced again before you go back to work. That way, when you come back, you are much more efficient.

Get Healthy NOW Action Steps:

• What thoughts do you find often running through your mind? Where do they come from? Are these thoughts truth? Right? Positive? Productive? Uplifting? List at least one way to re-frame this thought in a way that will be positive and productive.

_____

_____

_____

_____

_____

_____

_____

_____

_____

_____

_____

"Your body will manifest your thoughts both positive and negative. Don't think that you can get away with destructive thoughts but still have a healthy body."

-LeAnn Fritz

Words Are Important

The words we speak, both to ourselves and others, are powerful. It is essential to use positive language. Words such as "try" are negative and make you weaker. These words literally send a negative signal to the brain. These negative signals will ensure you fail, rather than build you up. Another powerful negative word is "can't". Often we use this term inaccurately. For example, "I just can't seem to get to work on time". The truth is that you are currently choosing to do other things with your time and aren't making it a priority. It's not that you physically can't get to work on time but rather that you won't get to work on time. Although this may sound harsh, it is critical to change this language because again, it sends a message to your brain to find ways to make you late. You can make incredible changes with ease once you use accurate, positive and powerful language.

Ask yourself this question, "How can I structure my life so I can be on time more often?" Your brain will seek an answer to that question. Give your brain the information it needs to make you successful.

• Do you find yourself using words and phrases like "I wish", "I hope", "I will try" or "I can't"? When do you say them? Upgrade those statements. Write them out here in a positive, true, and powerful way. (Ex: Instead of "I will try to get to work on time"...."Tomorrow I will set the alarm early and will get to work on time, feeling refreshed and ready to go!")

_____

_____

_____

_____

_____

_____

_____

_____

_____

_____

> *"Think twice before you speak, because your words and influence will plant the seed of either success or failure in the mind of another."*
>
> *-Napoleon Hill*

You're the Pilot

This may be a new concept for some but YOU have a lot of say about what goes on in your life. Too often we look to medical doctors, financial advisors, and other gurus for how to live our lives. Don't misunderstand. It's not that we shouldn't be talking to these people; it's that we should be using them as consultants rather than directors.

We ask questions and seek wisdom from others however, ultimately we have to do our homework and research what is best for ourselves. This may mean getting a second opinion, reading a book or asking more questions. Take one of my clients for example; before she came to me, she had sought the advice of a medical practitioner who recommended that she use a prescription diet pill. She really didn't think it was a good idea but ended up doing it anyway because it was what the doctor told her to do. Shortly after taking the pill she got light headed and dizzy, and then more side effects followed. So the question becomes, "Who is responsible for this?" My client is, NOT the doctor. I am not saying that doctors and other professionals are not responsible to make prudent recommendations. What I am saying is that no one is as responsible for your health as YOU are. It would have been wise for her to ask more questions, look up the medication, talk to the pharmacist and perhaps even get a second opinion before blindly following the doctor's advice. As the pilot, you still need others on your team, but you have the final say about how you choose to live.

Get Healthy NOW Action Steps

- List at least one area of your life where you are allowing others to make choices for you, even if/when the results aren't good. Why are you allowing this? List three actions that you can take to find a better solution.

_____

_____

_____

_____

_____

_____

_____

_____

_____

_____

Commit to Continuing Education

Becoming a lifelong learner is an essential part of being the best you! Your brain loves to learn, and the more you feed your brain good information, the better your brain will perform.

Often we think of continuing education in terms of going to conferences for your job yet it is so much more. For example, let's say you're in sales; how might your ability to close deals improve if you read one book per week about sales and client interactions? Or if you're a manager, what if you read one book per month or listened to management seminars regularly about how to manage your staff for improved efficiency and profit? Or, what if, regardless of what you do, you choose to read books about improving your diet? Do you think that would have a positive impact on your job, family and overall life? Of course! It doesn't matter what it is. The point here is to always be learning. You could hire a coach, go to a conference or retreat, read a book or watch a training video, the list is endless. Understand how you learn best and choose some great content to dive in to.

- List three areas of your life you would like to improve. For each one, list at least 3 ways of learning that could help that area, either directly (sales training for a person in sales) or indirectly (health information, health retreats/conferences for the same sales person). Now, circle one specific step that you can take action on TODAY!

_____

_____

_____

_____

_____

_____

_____

_____

_____

_____

_____

_____

_____

"You can make positive deposits in your own economy every day by reading and listening to powerful, positive, life-changing content and by associating with encouraging and hope-building people."
-Zig Ziglar

Set Goals and Write Them Down

Goals are the fuel that keeps us going when things don't go our way. They remind us what we are working for and keep us focused during our busy lives. They guide our priorities.

We often allow the fact that we don't have time to do that get in the way of setting goals. If you have time and would like to block out several hours to evaluate and set goals, that's great but isn't necessary. You can set goals anytime and anywhere. It doesn't take long. There are a couple of things to keep in mind. First, the goal must be specific and measurable. So instead of saying, "I want to close more clients this year", you might say, "I will have 50 new clients by Dec. 1st".

And your goal must have a deadline. This gives you a way to measure your success and then celebrate when you get there. Be flexible with yourself. If you need to adjust your goal, do it. It's okay. People who have goals get much more accomplished than those who don't, even if they don't reach those goals.

The final component of setting goals is that you have to <u>write them down</u>. Placing them in a prominent place is helpful so you are reminded of them regularly. As an added bonus to keep you motivated to work on your goals, tell a friend, family member, or co-worker who will keep you accountable and encourage you along the way. You will reach your goals. Start preparing for success!

• Record one goal for each of the following categories: Work, financial, personal, health, spiritual, family, and education (and other categories that may apply to you). Be specific and add a deadline. If you want to write out more goals later, great, but for now just do one for each. Then, under each one, list one simple step you can take to get started.

_____

_____

_____

_____

_____

_____

_____

_____

_____

_____

_____

_____

"The real value in setting goals is not in their achievement. The major reason for setting goals is to compel you to become the person it takes to achieve them."

-Jim Rohn

Self-Evaluation and Improvement

Like setting goals, this can take time, and doesn't have to be all-consuming. Where do you struggle? Where or with whom do you run into conflict or frustration? Where is your mind weak? All of these areas of improvement (notice I didn't say weaknesses), once improved, will have a huge impact on your life. For example, imagine if every day, you have conflict with a certain person at work that will affect your motivation at work, and also carry over into your life at home as you may come home feeling aggravated and irritable. But what if you recognize that you are not a victim and decide to develop new communication skills that change this relationship? Can you see how that would affect your productivity on the job, your relationships with your family, and perhaps even your health (by reducing stress and anxiety)?

We are holistic people and everything we do affects everything else. Think about the last time you were nervous and it caused your stomach to turn. Or the last time that you were embarrassed and felt your face turn red. Every thought and action has an effect. Where do you need to improve your thoughts or actions? If you can't think of areas that you need to improve, humble yourself and ask your coworkers, spouse, or a friend who will be honest with you.

- List 3 struggles, large or small. For each one, record how <u>you</u> may be contributing to them. Next, record what you may need to do to improve in this area (have a conversation, read a book, gain new skills, change your environment, remove the junk food from your kitchen, etc.).

_____

_____

_____

_____

_____

_____

_____

_____

_____

_____

_____

"You can make positive deposits into your own economy each day by reading and listening to life-changing content, and by associating with encouraging and hope-building people."

- Zig Ziglar

Read Daily

Reading every day gives you a mental workout, helps you learn and grow, improves your vocabulary and intellect, and also opens your eyes to new ways of thinking. If you aren't sure what to read, Google books on your favorite topics, such as "books about exercise", or "books about organizing your office, house or garage", etc. You can also get recommendations from your friends and coworkers. Find authors who you like and look up all the books they have written.

• If you don't already have one, create a list of books you want to read. If you don't know of specific books, then list categories (books about business, gardening, work life balance, natural health, etc). Find a comfortable place in your home or office that you will read each day. Choose the best time for you. You want this to be a time where you are alert and able to focus. Then simply schedule it in to your routine. It may be just 10 minutes each day to start and that is great. You can't read too much and the goal here is simply to create the habit.

Visualize Daily

Visualization is similar to setting goals. It doesn't have to be a long, formal process. So often we don't take time to even think about what we want, let alone picture it. It's easy. Get a picture in your mind of what you want. It could be a promotion at work, a certain level of health, a happy marriage or anything else that is important to you. Picture it coming easily and with joy. Now block out at least one minute in the morning and one minute before you go to sleep to allow your mind to focus on this concept or image. If you have time and are feeling ambitious, you can take this to the next level by creating a vision board. This is where you draw or cut out pictures that represent what you want to achieve and put them on a poster board (or whatever you want them on). The vision board creates a literal visual reminder to your subconscious mind regarding what you are working toward.

Get Healthy NOW Action Steps

- Decide something that you want to achieve. It could be in any category (like, health, business/career, financial, academic, family or others). Briefly write out what your vision is for this goal. Now, put a reminder next to your bed that reminds you to pause for one minute each morning and night to do this exercise. Once you have placed the reminder near your bed, sign your name at the bottom of this page as a sign of commitment to take action

_____

_____

_____

_____

_____

_____

_____

_____

_____

_____

Positive Environment

A positive and healthy environment is something that you can influence to help you get more out of your day.

Your environment has many components. First, think about what you hear. Whenever possible, eliminate "noise pollution" that annoys or distracts you. Put up curtains (to deaden the sound a bit) or just add soft music. If possible and appropriate, it may help to wear sound deadening headphones with music that help you concentrate and focus.

What do you see? Is there clutter everywhere? Perhaps you could place a simple positive quote near your workstation or a picture of your loved ones.

How about what you smell? Are there the smells of tempting foods (that you don't want to eat)? Is there a musty smell? Could you open windows or use essential oils to improve this?

What about the people you are around? Are they generally positive and uplifting? If so, great! If not, can you spend less time with them? If not, how do you need to think differently in order to stay energized in this environment? What other factors contribute to your environment? What about yourself, do you make the atmosphere better or worse for yourself and others?

- Evaluate your environment at work or at home (whichever you want to focus on first). What do you hear? What do you see? Smell? What are the people like? Other factors? Now, next to each category, brain storm at least one simple way that YOU can improve your surroundings.

_____

_____

_____

_____

_____

_____

_____

_____

_____

_____

_____

Priorities

Your priorities reflect your values. In every case, your priorities can be seen not in what you say, but in how you live.

Please allow me to give you an example from my own life. I spend a lot of money on my health. I buy all organic food, I go to a holistic dentist, take supplements, invest in health and detox retreats, and much more. Sometimes clients will tell me that they can't afford to eat organic. My answer is always the same. You can't afford NOT to eat organic. The payoff is much more than just money. I would drive an older car, live in a smaller house and never go out to eat before I would give up my health investments. Why? Is it because I am obsessed with perfect health? No! It's because everything else is irrelevant if I lost my abundant and optimal health. Being healthy for me is FREEDOM. It helps me get more out of relationships, business and life in general.

What good is a nice car and big house and fancy date nights if I am sick or not feeling well to enjoy them? It would all mean nothing. Because of my great energy and productivity, I am able to give of myself in my business, in my church, and at home without feeling run down. This is just one example. Please understand, this is not to say that you shouldn't have nice things. It just serves as an illustration of priorities. If you feel that you "can't afford organic food" consider where you could cut expenses: do you drive expensive cars, pay for cable TV, eat out often or spend thousands of dollars each year on gifts, landscaping or other things where you could save money, freeing up more funds to invest in your health?

This principle could apply to time with your family, financial investments, tasks at work, and really anything. Have priorities that guide your decisions. This can also work on another scale, such as buying/drinking less coffee each week and putting the difference that you would save toward your higher priority. For example, if you usually spend $5/weekday on a fancy coffee, if you started doing that just one day/week instead of five, you would have an extra $80 per month to put toward your higher priority. Or, if you work late every night but miss your family, once a week, leave work early, ignore the house work and go on a date or play with your kids/nieces/ nephews/grandkids, or whatever fits your priorities.

Get Healthy NOW Action Steps

- According to the way you are living, where do your priorities need to be shaped or changed? Health? Family? Finances? Work-life balance? What are some principles that will shape those priorities? List at least one action step for each category that you could take to create more consistency with what you want your life to reflect.

_____

_____

_____

_____

_____

_____

_____

_____

_____

_____

_____

Car College

Turn your car time into learning time. This is a great time to listen to audios about anything that you want to learn more about. It could be personal development and motivation, health and stress management, training that is specific to improving your job or an encouraging message from your pastor. This way, you will arrive (wherever you are going) inspired, encouraged and excited about what you just learned. You can also feel good about "redeeming" the otherwise wasted car time.

If you can spare a moment before you get out of your car, write something down about whatever you were listening to. It can be something that you learned or an action step you want to take. There is power in the written word. Just like when you write out your goals, the commitment level goes up.

Get Healthy NOW Action Steps

• How much time do you spend in your car each week? What do you want to learn? Who do you love to learn from? Where can you purchase or rent (library) these audios? Make a list of topics and choose one that you will get right away.

_____

_____

_____

_____

_____

_____

_____

_____

_____

_____

Genetics Loads the Gun, You Pull the Trigger

It's time to think differently about our genetics. Genetics load the gun, but you pull the trigger. You are not doomed by the health issues and habits of your parents or grandparents. Often what we assume is genetic is actually environmental and even more often a specific choice. If you live similar to how your parents lived, your chances of having similar issues increases. Genetics do indeed load the gun...so you may indeed have a weakness or tendency, however that doesn't mean that you will get sick, it just means that you may have to work a little harder in that specific area. Remember the hope that we gain when we take full responsibility for our choices and circumstances.

- What have you believed about yourself because of your genetics/ family? Do you think that you're just overweight? Depressed? Or pre-destined for cancer, diabetes, or heart disease? Record a powerful statement here. Put it in your own words, but something along the lines of..."I have the power to choose how I live, and I choose to live healthy rather than diabetic like my father."

_____

_____

_____

_____

_____

_____

_____

_____

_____

_____

_____

_____

"Genetics loads the gun, you pull the trigger."
-Gabriel Cousens

Emotions

Emotions color our world and keep things interesting. However negative emotions can cause great harm over time. Specific negative emotions also have an affinity for harming specific organs.

Here are some examples: Fear paralyzes us mentally, diminishes creativity, and weakens the kidneys. We live in a fear-based culture. We are afraid to fail and afraid to succeed. Afraid to look stupid. Afraid that we won't fit in. Medical doctors, the government and many others use fear to motivate us to do what they would have us do.

Anger affects the blood pressure, muscles, and liver.
Bitterness affects our relationships with others and our gall bladder.
Grief and sadness tend to bring us low, reducing confidence and causing problems in the lungs.

So what is the lesson? Ultimately in order to have a clear mind, we need to stay on top of these negative emotions and not allow them to gain momentum. It is okay and even normal to experience these emotions, we just don't want to let them get out of control before we take action. An important part of this is determining to have current and proper communication in relationships. If you are upset with someone or have been hurt by someone, work it out by talking to them as soon as possible rather than waiting until there is a major blow up. One must be able to express hurts and feelings to those they are having issues with. Forgiveness is also critical to emotional wellness and balance. When these things are addressed, your mind is clearer and free to focus on more important things such as your family, job or education.

Get Healthy NOW Action Steps

• Are there any negative emotions that you are regularly feeling? Where are they coming from? How have you contributed to or fed into them? List three things that you can do to up-root these issues now.

_____

_____

_____

_____

_____

_____

_____

_____

_____

_____

_____

Gifts

Everything is a gift, even the trials of life. Develop the skill of seeing the gift in the struggle. In everything, there is some diamond in the rough. Perhaps it's a lesson to be learned, or something to be grateful for that you had lost sight of. When we begin to see our circumstances in this light it takes us out of having a victim mentality and restores our hope. Nothing happens randomly or because of "bad luck"; rather everything is to help you grow and expand in some area of life where you currently have an area needing improvement.

- List 3 trials that you are currently facing (big or small). Next to each one, record at least one gift that you could potentially be receiving through that struggle. How does this view change your perspective?

_____

_____

_____

_____

_____

_____

_____

_____

_____

_____

_____

Guard Your Eyes and Ears

Be careful what you let into your mind through the gates of your eyes and ears. In terms of your eyes, avoid watching television, movies, and other such things that invoke fear, sadness or other negative emotions. This will be different for different people but violent TV, movies, and news would be examples of this. As for your ears, the same is true. Listen to radio/audios that are uplifting. Be careful not to listen to lots of negative talk or gossip. Your mind is not a garbage can so don't let other people put their trash in it. What you watch (and listen to) on TV and movies can be a great example of many negative messages that will start to permeate your mind. Messages such as "rich people are greedy", "marriage is disposable" and "all teenagers are selfish" can start to shape our thinking about life in a negative way that is also inaccurate.

- Are you currently watching anything that causes you to lose sleep
  or clutters your mind with negative images? Why? What do you love
  about it and how could you satisfy that desire some other way? What
  about your ears? What are you listening to that is not helping you stay
  clear and focused? Again, why? List a "next step" for each one. What
  commitment can you make to guard your brain?

_____

_____

_____

_____

_____

_____

_____

_____

_____

_____

_____

_____

"Your mind is not a garbage can so don't let other people put their trash in it."

-LeAnn Fritz

Invite Feedback

Be teachable and humble. How we handle constructive (or not so constructive) criticism says a lot about us and our desire to really grow and expand into the best we can possibly be. When you get feedback from someone, mine it for gold. Even if you don't agree with 98% of it, that 2% might be exactly what you needed to hear to have an understanding of what you need to work on and change. This is true at work, in your family, and also in other groups that you are part of. Seek not to take it personally, but rather use it for your benefit and growth. In most cases, people mean it to be helpful, but even if they don't, it can still be used to launch you to the next level.

To take it to the next level ASK for feedback. Ask your co-workers to tell you one specific thing that you could do better in your next presentation. Ask your spouse how you could be a better husband/wife. Ask your kids how you could be a better mom/dad. Ask your Team Leader at work what you would need to improve to be promoted to the next level. Strive for excellence!

• Briefly describe the last time you were criticized or you received feedback. How did you respond to the person? How did you feel internally? What do you need to change for next time? If you want to get to the next level even faster, ask a trusted friend, family member, or coworker what they see that you most need to improve. Who could you ask for feedback? Just be ready to grow!

_____

_____

_____

_____

_____

_____

_____

_____

_____

_____

_____

_____

"A man must be big enough to admit his mistakes, smart enough to profit from them, and strong enough to correct them."
-John Maxwell

Failure...is There Such a Thing?

You only have a complete failure if you don't learn anything. So when you perceive that you have failed, don't quit. Ask yourself, "What is the lesson here for me?" If you can't think of anything, ask someone to help you think it through. For example, let's say that you have made a goal to exercise 5 days per week for a month. After two weeks of doing great, things get busy and you miss two work outs. Is this a failure? For some, perhaps, because they would throw away the entire program since they got off track. Instead, what if you learned that you may need to have a backup plan for a shorter workout on those extra busy days? And then you follow it up by getting right back on track the next day with your regular routine. Don't throw away progress at the hand of perfection. Small steps add up over time. The principle of learning from our "failures" gives us hope to keep going and redeems what would otherwise be a pointless frustration. When we see these failures as an opportunity to learn, they become a gift (as mentioned in a previous tip) rather than a point of despair. Although you can't turn back time, or undo the past, you can always take action now in some positive direction.

- Record at least one area where you feel you have failed. Write down at least 2 things that you could learn from this experience. Then record three next steps to get back on track.

_____

_____

_____

_____

_____

_____

_____

_____

_____

_____

_____

_____

> *"I've come to believe that all my past failure and frustration were actually laying the foundation for the understandings that have created the new level of living I now enjoy."*
>
> *-Tony Robbins*

Ask Good Questions of Yourself

When you ask yourself good questions, your brain will give you good answers. For example, if you rehearse questions like, "What am I missing? How can I support my body and help it release weight in a healthy way? What COULD I do to lose weight?" Your brain will likely explode with answers, such as "find a friend to exercise with", "get more rest", "balance hormones", "eat more vegetables", "go seek help from a detox specialist", "eat less at night", and many more factors that can contribute to holding onto extra weight. However, the opposite is also true.

When you ask yourself bad questions, you get bad answers. For instance, if you keep saying to yourself, "why can't I lose weight"...your brain produces answers that validate the implied outcome that you indeed can't lose weight. You may come up with answers like, "because you're genetically heavy", or "because you're addicted to food", or "because your job/marriage/family creates too much stress".

Next time you feel challenged, frame your questions in a positive light. It sets your brain into action and gets it working for you even when you aren't thinking about it.

- List three challenges that you are currently facing. For each one, write out at least one positive, solution-oriented question. Then, jot down the answers that automatically come to mind.

_____

_____

_____

_____

_____

_____

_____

_____

_____

_____

_____

_____

"Successful people ask better questions, and as a result, they get better answers."

-Tony Robbins

Slow and Steady Wins the Race

The goal of this book is to help you make changes about what you put in your mind, your body, and your life in order to help you create more energy, better productivity, and ultimately, a more amazing YOU! The goal is slow, sustainable changes over the long haul. For example, if you drink a pot of coffee every day, it is probably not sustainable to eliminate coffee altogether overnight. Instead, start by adding more water and then reducing your coffee by 10-20% each week for the next several weeks. This is change that will last and won't be so hard on your body, mind, or spirit in the meantime.

The rate at which you choose to progress will depend on your personality and comfort level to some degree. However, know that all change can be uncomfortable at first so don't be alarmed or necessarily think that you are moving too quickly if you feel like you're struggling at first. If you have a strong motivation to make radical changes quickly, do so, but just be sure that you support your holistic self so that you can sustain the change. Think of lifestyle rather than diet.

Get Healthy NOW Action Steps

- List 5 things that you want to change (in any area: health, work, finances, family, spiritual, etc.). What do you want the long-term result to look like? What are the baby steps in between that will help you get there. List one for each thing you want to change.

_____

_____

_____

_____

_____

_____

_____

_____

_____

_____

_____

_____

"Little hinges swing big doors."

-W. Clement Stone

- 47 -

Section 2 – What You Put in Your Body

What you put in your BODY will help your energy, productivity, and YOU. Certain foods will make you tired and will cloud your thinking making it difficult to concentrate. On the other hand, there is a wide variety of delicious and amazing whole fresh foods that will help you to look and feel amazing, full of energy and able to think clearly and make good decisions quickly. Which will you choose? This section will give you tools to re-build your body cell by cell in a way that you will hardly believe the transformation. Start now!

Water

Drink more water. Ideally, sip it all day long, starting first thing in the morning. Dehydration is the NUMBER ONE cause of mid-day fatigue. It is also the leading reason for high blood pressure. Water is needed for EVERY function in the human body. If you consume lots of sugar, processed/white table salt, alcohol or caffeine, you will need even MORE water as these tend to dehydrate your body.

It is vital to get clean pure water, such as distilled or reverse osmosis. City water is especially harmful as it is often full of chemicals, medications and bacteria. Well water is usually better but it would be wise to have it tested to be sure. Many bottled waters have added minerals that are synthetic. Avoid water with any ingredients besides "water". If you get sick of plain water, add fresh lemon or lime juice (you can add a small amount of natural sweetener if desired).

Roughly estimated, you should consume about half your weight in ounces. For example, if you weigh 200 lbs, you will need approximately 100 oz. of water per day. Of course this number will vary from person to person depending on your climate, activity level and nutrition/diet. The brain is made primarily of fat and water, so you if are even mildly dehydrated, you will struggle to think clearly and have optimal mental energy. This can effect your work, family relationships and more...such a simple fix! Go fill your water bottle and start sipping!

- What is your next step? How much water are you currently drinking? How much will you commit to drinking this week? What do you need to do to help yourself consume more water? Do you need to buy a water bottle? Put a reminder on your phone to take a drink every 30 minutes? Look for a good place to buy water? Perhaps it would help to get a large container that will fit your daily requirements in it and fill it each morning to see how you are doing. Record at least one action step here.

_____

_____

_____

_____

_____

_____

_____

_____

_____

Organic Food is Safer and Has More Minerals Than Conventionally Grown/Raised Food

This is important for two reasons. First, when you eat chemicals such as pesticides, herbicides, fertilizers, hormones, and antibiotics, you are consuming many carcinogenic (cancer causing) substances. These may not cause an immediate problem, but over time they will accumulate and cause inflammation, excess weight, a tired, sluggish mind, and eventually can lead to disease.

The other factor to consider is that when you are eating conventionally grown foods, it can be difficult to meet your nutritional needs because the food is so depleted. You will find yourself over eating because although your stomach is full, your cells still have nutritional needs that aren't being addressed. If you can't buy ALL organic, start with the most important foods, the ones that are most contaminated with chemicals. Buy organic: All animal products (meat, dairy, eggs), all greens (spinach, kale, romaine, etc.), all berries, cherries, apples, corn, and soy. Foods that are less critical to buy organic: bananas, citrus, avocados, broccoli, asparagus, and pineapple.

Also, because of the lack of mineral content in the food of non-organic food, it tends to have more bitterness. Compare the taste of organic raw celery or spinach to conventionally grown. In many cases, I have had client tell me that they don't like spinach for example. However they find when they buy it organic, they do indeed like it.

• What foods do you eat the most from the list that you should buy organic? Where can you find them?

_____

_____

_____

_____

_____

_____

_____

_____

_____

_____

_____

"Nearly every function of the body requires water. Nothing living thrives without water...this includes YOU."

-LeAnn Fritz

Eat More Greens

Dark leafy greens are some of the most nutrient dense foods that you can consume. They are loaded with minerals, vitamins, and various other nutrients that the body needs, and yet have very few calories. Some examples of dark leafy greens are kale, spinach, romaine, chard, watercress, and arugula. Minerals are needed in abundance for proper body functions. Minerals are used up quickly when you are lacking sleep, under a great deal of stress, or if you are working out regularly. Greens can be eaten in salads, green smoothies, green juices, green powders, or chopped up into soups or steamed vegetables. These foods should be part of your daily diet and will help to increase your energy and stamina a great deal. Greens are heavily sprayed with the contaminants mentioned in the previous tip, so choose organic when you shop.

• What dishes do you LOVE that contain greens? How can you make them a bigger part of your diet? If you don't care for them or haven't tried many greens, you may want to sneak them in by finely chopping them and adding to foods that you are already eating.

_____

_____

_____

_____

_____

_____

_____

_____

_____

_____

_____

"Eating organic supports the healing process. Non-organic foods contain pesticides and various chemicals that undermine the body's effort to repair."

-LeAnn Fritz

Fat

Eating healthy fats is a great way to help your brain function optimally. Healthy fats coat the myelin sheaths of the nerves, as well as fuel the brain. This combination will help you feel efficient and calm so that you can balance all of the many things that you need to accomplish, both at work and at home.

Your brain is made primarily of water and fat so those are primary fuels for optimal thinking, clarity and mental calmness. As a side benefit, healthy fats can also make you feel full as well as decrease excess weight. The best fats to include are raw organic walnuts, raw organic sunflower seeds, flax seeds, chia seeds, hemp seeds and avocados. Avocados and hemp seeds are wonderful in salads. The other fats can be added to oatmeal, smoothies or yogurts. Don't confuse these fats with UNhealthy fats such as hydrogenated oils, fried foods, canola oil, and highly heated fats (like in potato chips), just to name a few. These fats are extremely harmful to the body and specifically to the liver and gall bladder.

- Take inventory of your pantry. Do you have healthy fats on hand? If not, make your shopping list. How can you add these fats to your regular routine?

Raw Foods

Raw foods (sometimes referred to as live foods) are all plant based specifically, fruits, vegetables, seeds, nuts, grains, beans, sprouts and legumes. This does not include raw meat, cheese or eggs.

Eating more raw foods greatly increases your energy and vitality in several ways. One of the most important is that raw foods provide more nutrition. Many nutrients are heat sensitive. Protein for example is reduced by about 50% when cooked. Many other vitamins and minerals are lost as well, up to 90% when heated. This means that you may need to eat two to three times more food (cooked) to get the amount of nutrition that your body needs for optimal function.

Another key benefit is that raw foods are easier to digest (assuming that you chew properly and thoroughly). Live or raw foods have enough enzymes in them to digest themselves. For example, if you eat a salad or smoothie loaded with raw plant based ingredients, you will usually have good digestion for that meal. However if you eat a meal of only cooked or processed foods, your body is forced to dip into your reserves for enough enzymes to digest that meal. Raw foods are easier to digest, so more of your energy can be used to complete other tasks at work or at home.

This would be no problem in many cultures, however here in the United States, because so much of our food source is cooked and processed, most Americans have completely depleted their enzyme stores by the age of 25 years. For the average American, about 80% of one's total energy is used to digest food. This is mainly because of the number of difficult to digest foods we eat. Seek to eat raw foods with each meal. Perhaps make one meal per day completely raw such as a large salad or a green smoothie.

• How can you add more raw foods to your diet? Do you love fruit salad for dessert? Could you flavor your oatmeal with raw walnuts, cinnamon and a chopped apple instead of processed sugar? What are your favorite nuts? Fruits? Vegetables? How can you get more of these in each day? Make at least one meal per day totally raw (salad, smoothie, guacamole with vegetables, etc.) or have some raw food with each meal. Which would work best for you?

_____

_____

_____

_____

_____

_____

_____

_____

_____

_____

Superfoods
Superfoods are foods that contain an unusually high amount of nutrients. Some of these foods are delicious just eaten plain while others are often blended into a smoothie or even made into a tea.

Many superfoods have specific adaptogenic properties, meaning they balance body systems that are either under or over active. For example, maca, is a root that is commonly ground into a powder and added to smoothies, puddings and other foods. It tends to increase energy and stamina, as well as balance hormones. Goji berries are another wonderful superfood. Goji berries are low glycemic (so they won't spike your blood sugar). They are chewy and sweet and go well in trail mix, on cereals, or sprinkled over desserts of any kind. Goji berries tend to increase energy, as well as improve mental clarity. For overall wellness and detoxification, chlorella can be helpful. If you need more protein, spirulina is the best. Chia and hemp seeds are both good sources of protein and fat. Chia has lots of calcium as well. Cacao is raw unprocessed chocolate and is loaded with magnesium. Just be sure that no matter which superfoods you choose, it is important to get them from a pure, raw organic source.

Get Healthy NOW Action Steps

- What is lacking in your health? Is there a specific condition that you would like to work on? Which superfoods would you LOVE to add? If you need help here, see the resource section at the back of the book.

_____

_____

_____

_____

_____

_____

_____

_____

_____

_____

Supplements

Many people struggle with the thought of taking supplements. However, there are several factors to consider for why supplementation is helpful and even necessary. First, there are several elements such as poor food quality (foods that contain processed sugars, highly heated fats, chemicals, dyes, or pesticides), increased stress, and toxicity in the air that are all at an all-time high, which increases our need to supplement. This is another reason why it is so important to move toward the majority of your food coming from whole, natural plant based sources as these foods help to counter the negative effects from some of the other toxicity that we are faced with.

An additional key factor when it comes to supplements is to be sure that you are getting really pure and effective supplements without any fillers or excipients that will cause harm to the body. Do not choose the cheapest ones you can find, and avoid those at your local big box stores and pharmacies as they tend to use a lot of cheap fillers and low quality ingredients.

Studies continually show that Americans are deficient in nearly <u>every</u> nutrient. Literally! Consider that every nutrient has multiple functions in the body and you begin to understand why there are so many health issues in the United States. It is ideal to go to a natural health practitioner and talk to them about what you specifically will need for your body. However, in the meantime, it is great to start with a greens powder, plant based digestive enzymes, B12, minerals, DHA, and a pro-biotic.

These are, of course, in addition to a healthy diet, a lot of water, good sleep and other basic health habits. Supplements are just that, SUPPLEMENTS. They should supplement, rather than take the place of an overall healthy life style. For more information about how to access the most effective supplements, see the resource section in the back of this book.

- Before supplementing, what basic health habits do you need to improve? List 3 here. Now choose the one that may have the highest impact. List the top three supplements that you believe would be helpful for you. If you aren't sure, your next step is to find a natural health practitioner who has a great understanding of nutrition. After some basic simple testing, they should be able to guide you specifically on what will work best for you and your body.

"There is no supplement to take the place of drinking water, deep breathing, eating healthy food and exercise"

-LeAnn Fritz

Green Smoothies

Green smoothies are a wonderful addition to your daily routine and are easy to make for your whole family. They can be made quickly; they taste great and can be adjusted to your liking in terms of taste, nutritional needs, and consistency.

Green smoothies are an awesome way to get more dark leafy greens into your body without having to chew them. Put into your blender just four simple ingredients: Dark leafy greens (organic spinach, kale, romaine, chard), healthy fat (about 2-4 Tbls. coconut oil, or hemp, chia or flax seeds, or 1/2 avocado), liquid (water, coconut, rice or almond milk), and fresh or frozen fruit (whatever you like). Blend and taste test. Adjust as needed...if it's not sweet enough, add more fruit or a tablespoon of raw honey or real maple syrup or a few drops of liquid stevia...if it's too thick, add more liquid etc.

The greens give lots of fiber, vitamins and minerals, as well as chlorophyll, which is a wonderful blood purifier. The fat helps the brain and nervous system function optimally and also helps the smoothie stick with you longer. The liquid is mainly just to help the blender work. The better your blender, the less you will need. The fruit offers fiber, vitamins and minerals, and is the main flavor of your smoothie. If you aren't using frozen fruit, you may want to add a few ice cubes. You can also add superfoods or superfood powders such as greens powders, plant based protein powders, maca, or goji berries (soak for 30 minutes before using) to your smoothie.

Replacing one meal per day with a green smoothie would be a big step toward increasing your energy and getting more done. You just get so much good nutritional bang for your caloric buck with these.

- Make a list of anything you need to get started. Do you have a good blender? For more information about getting an incredible blender, see the resource section at the back of the book. Is your kitchen stocked with greens, fruit, and some healthy fats? When is the best time for you to make this (breakfast, lunch or dinner)? Do you want to add any extras (for example if you work out hard, you may want to add some high quality plant based protein powder)? If so, list it here.

_____

_____

_____

_____

_____

_____

_____

_____

_____

_____

_____

_____

"If you make no other changes, but add a green smoothie as one meal per day, you will initiate an incredible cascade effect of positive changes in your health and life."

-LeAnn Fritz

Whole Foods

Whole foods grow from the earth and have not been processed in any way. The goal is to make the majority of your diet from whole foods. This gives us a massive variety of fruits, vegetable, nuts, seeds, beans, lentils, and whole grains. So for example, oats are a whole food. When you highly heat oats and then combine them with hydrogenated oils, sugar, dyes and other preservatives to make a frosted cereal for example, they are no longer a whole food.

There are literally hundreds of delicious combinations of whole foods. It can seem intimidating at first, but keep it simple and take it one new food at a time. Let's choose lentils for example. They are a great source of fiber and protein but don't have a strong flavor so they tend to just blend into whatever you put them with. Cook up a batch of lentils, then just add them to things that you are already eating to increase the protein, fiber, and fullness factor. Add a 1/2 c. of cooked lentils to your salad, soups, mashed potatoes, stir fry, wrap or taco. You can do the same things with beans, hemp seeds, and avocados. The great thing is you don't necessarily have to come up with "new recipes/meals", but rather just add more healthy whole foods to your current diet.

Eventually, all of the tasty whole foods will have you feeling so energetic that some of the less nutritious foods will just get crowded out. If you love to cook or prepare food, by all means, start experimenting. But if you don't, just add more whole foods to your current meals.

Get Healthy NOW Action Steps

- Make a list of a few of your favorite whole foods from each category (fruits, veggies, beans, lentils, nuts and seeds). If your kitchen isn't stocked with them, get to the grocery store with this list and stock up. Choose at least one "new" food that you will experiment with (beans, lentils, pine nuts, hemp seeds, whole grains-such as oats or quinoa, etc.). List at least 3 things that you currently eat that you could add them to.

_____

_____

_____

_____

_____

_____

_____

_____

_____

_____

Lemon/Lime Water in the Morning

Starting your day with lemon or lime water is a great way to re-hydrate, add minerals, and begin with a natural gentle cleansing for the body. Take half of a lemon or lime and squeeze it into a quart of water. If you like it sweeter, like a lemon- or lime-aid, add about 10 drops of liquid stevia. If you don't have blood sugar issues, you can use 1 teaspoon of raw honey or real maple syrup instead. For those in a cold climate, you can use hot or warm water to make a lemon tea. After 8 hours or more of not drinking (during the night), the body will use this drink to help flush out toxins that may have been released into the blood stream while you were sleeping, but still haven't been eliminated from the body.

Get Healthy Now Action Steps

- Gather your lemons or limes, a mason jar, good water and a natural sweetener and set them in the kitchen. As soon as you get up in the morning, make the drink and enjoy. List here three reasons why you want to do this natural detoxification drink. You tend to get more out of something when you have a goal or intension.

_____

_____

_____

_____

_____

_____

_____

_____

_____

_____

_____

"Lemon or lime water each morning is a critical part of daily detoxification."

-LeAnn Fritz

Decrease Meat

Decrease means decrease, not eliminate. First, let me define meat as the flesh of any animal, including cow, deer, pig, sheep, chicken, turkey, fish, etc. If you love meat, eat it. Just know what you are eating and seek to eat less of it.

Meat is really difficult to digest. For this reason, it tends to literally rot in the stomach, often creating digestive disturbances. It is also acidic which can lead to a great deal of pain and inflammation in the body over time. If you are already dealing with any sort of pain or inflammatory conditions, eat very little, if any meat.

What about protein? Meat does contain protein, but because the structure of it makes it so difficult to digest and use, you actually get very little protein from meat per calorie as compared to spirulina, chlorella, kale, beans, lentils, hemp seeds and spinach, with a much smaller toxic load for the body to contend with. Black bean burgers, vegan bean dips, lentil soups and quinoa burgers are also delicious options.

Animal flesh holds toxins at levels several times greater than plants so that means that any toxic feed or metabolic toxins in the animal will be trapped in its flesh. If you prefer to eat meat, buy local, organic, fresh, free-range/grass-fed cuts from farmers who you know and trust. Less meat will give your digestion a break and you will have more energy for other things.

• What are some healthier substitutes that you could use to replace some of the meat that you are eating? How could you incorporate this into your daily routine? One example would be to make chili with little to no meat, but instead, extra beans, lentils and vegetables.

_____

_____

_____

_____

_____

_____

_____

_____

_____

_____

_____

"Protein does not equal meat."

-LeAnn Fritz

Decrease Dairy

Dairy is any product made from cow's milk. This would include most conventional milks, cheeses, yogurts, ice cream and cheese flavored snacks like chips and crackers.

It is estimated that about 80% of the population is allergic to dairy. This allergy will often manifest in subtle ways, such as decreased immunity, increased digestive issues, sinus trouble, and overall more mucous production. Cow's milk was actually designed for baby cows. Calves come out weighing about 150 pounds and have four stomachs. Can you see how we, and our little ones, have a hard time digesting these things?

Cow's milk also has a great concentration of toxins, including pus cells, hormones, antibiotics and various other bacteria. Don't worry...there are lots of delicious alternatives. Coconut milk, almond milk and rice milk are all wonderful and they come in chocolate, vanilla and plain. They are easy to make yourself if you're interested. You can also buy yogurts, cheeses and ice creams made from these delicious alternatives. If you really strongly prefer dairy, buy organic. If you can find local and organic, that would be even better. Avoid soy...more to come on that.

- List your favorite dairy products. What do you like about them? How could that desire be satisfied with other foods? For example, if you love ranch dressing because it's creamy, you could make a dressing with spices and an avocado base that would also be creamy but much healthier. Choose some healthy dairy alternatives to test out today in your kitchen.

Decrease Caffeine

Caffeine is really congesting to your liver and especially beats up on your adrenal glands. The liver impacts your mood, hormones, digestion and your body's ability to filter toxins. When your adrenals are overworked and stressed it will impact your energy level, your hormones and your ability to properly handle stress. Caffeine tends to give you a short term sense of false energy and then a crash.

Caffeine is commonly found in high quantities in coffee and soda. The important question to ask here is why you drink caffeine. If it's because you like the taste of coffee or pop, that is less of an issue because it isn't difficult to find other drinks that have a taste you enjoy. For example, if you drink coffee, try an herbal coffee made of chicory and other herbs. Instead of soda, try Izze's or Kombucha (these options are at most health food stores). However, if it's because you need a kick to get going or keep going, that is a different issue. It is important to figure out why you need the kick. We aren't tired because we have a coffee, soda or caffeine deficiency. We are tired because we are nutrient deficient or overall depleted and out of balance.

- How many servings of caffeine are you currently drinking each day? Why do you drink it? What would help decrease your need for it? Do you need to get more sleep? Are you eating too much sugar that is causing your energy to crash? Do you eat a lot of processed foods? Are you dehydrated? List three actions that you can ADD to your routine that will help you taper off caffeine. A few examples might be: go to bed by 10 PM, drink lemon water in the morning, drink herbal tea, eat more whole foods, etc.

_____

_____

_____

_____

_____

_____

_____

_____

_____

_____

"Your body is a high performance machine and the only one you get. You wouldn't put coffee in the tank of your car. Why? Because it was designed to run on a specific fuel. So was your body. Give it what it was designed to run on. It will in turn give you optimal performance."

-LeAnn Fritz

Decrease Processed Foods

Processed foods are loaded with anti-nutrients. That is things that create more work and stress in the body and rob your body of any nutrient reserves. Highly heated oils, chemical flavors and colors, sugar, corn and soy products, and preservatives such as MSG in processed foods and are all contributors to the toxic load in the body which translates to low energy and decreased productivity.

These foods were created to be shelf stable for long periods of time. They are often highly addicting, which is why it's hard to quit eating them. These are NOT whole foods. Some examples would be crackers, chips, breads, cookies, canned foods and candy bars. Most products that come in a can, bag or box are processed. You can also get a good idea by looking at the ingredients. If there are words that you don't know or a long list of ingredients, the chances are pretty high that you are looking at a processed food.

These foods also give a false sense of energy, followed by a long crash. They often have neuro-toxins, also referred to as excitotoxins (such as MSG) that disturb the brain's neurotransmitters and cause a person to lose focus, as well as brain cells. Often these foods are eaten because they are fast and convenient. But what is faster than an apple or a handful of nuts?

• What processed foods do you eat daily? Why do you eat them? Taste? Convenience? Social reasons? Laziness? List several alternatives that you could take to replace some of these foods.

_____

_____

_____

_____

_____

_____

_____

_____

_____

_____

_____

Eat Sweets, but Not Sugar!

The sweet taste in your mouth is not the problem; it's the massive amounts of processed sugar. There are several harmful sweeteners to avoid including Splenda, white and brown sugar, high fructose corn syrup, aspartame and Nutrasweet, to name a few. These are mainly in pre-packaged, processed foods, so if you are eating mostly whole foods, you won't need to worry about this as much.

These sugars spike the blood sugar, harm the brain, pancreas and liver and over time can cause serious health problems. They also feed infection and hinder the immune system. One of the best sweeteners to use that won't spike your blood sugars at all is stevia. Stevia is a plant. It comes in a green powder form and also in a liquid. It is way sweeter than sugar so you only need a tiny amount and if you get too much it tastes bitter. Xylitol, (from birch, not corn) is another low glycemic (doesn't raise the blood sugar) sweetener. You can also use chopped or crushed fresh fruit, dried fruits, raw honey, agave nectar, yacon syrup and pure maple syrup. In oatmeal, for example, instead of using brown sugar, try chopped fresh fruit. In baking, use honey, maple syrup, xylitol or stevia (depending on what you are making).

When you upgrade your sweeteners, you get more minerals with much less crash. If you are diabetic or sensitive to sugar, stick with fresh berries, stevia or xylitol. Sweeteners like raw honey and maple syrup are much better than sugar but do still raise your blood sugar.

• Where do you get sugar in your diet? Cereal? Oatmeal? Ice cream? Candy? Sodas? How can you upgrade by making your own treats or adding an alternative sweetener?

_____

_____

_____

_____

_____

_____

_____

_____

_____

_____

_____

"It's wise to avoid sugar, not sweetness."

-LeAnn Fritz

Use Good Salt

There is a big difference between white table salt and sun dried pink Himalayan salt. White table salt is toxic to the body. It increases water retention, thickens the blood (forcing the heart to work harder to pump blood to the extremities), increases blood pressure, and hinders digestion. Even if you don't add a lot of salt to your diet if you're eating lots of fast food, processed food, or other pre-packaged foods, you are probably getting a great deal of harmful salt. Cheese, processed meats, TV dinners, soups and potato chips are especially high in poor quality salt.

There is a very simple four-part remedy to flushing this type of salt out of the body. First, eliminate or dramatically reduce your intake of harmful salt. There is no point in flushing it out if you're still ingesting it. Second, increase your water intake. Third, increase foods that have natural sodium, such as celery, kale, spinach and sea vegetables. Finally, add good, healthy, mineral-rich salt into your diet. Good salt will never be white, but rather pink, gray or light brown (sand-colored). It should be sun dried rather than processed with high heat. This type of salt will not make you feel bloated or swollen. It will give minerals to the body and is especially helpful after a workout where you are losing salt in perspiration. Carry good salt with you in your car, purse or in a baggie in your pocket when you are going to be eating out so it is always on hand and you aren't tempted to use regular table salt.

- List where you are currently getting poor quality salt on a regular basis? How can you replace those items with healthier salts? For example, although homemade soup is best, if you must buy canned soup, get salt free and then add your own good salt. If eating out a lot is part of your life, ask for items without salt and then bring your own to add. Also, if you know that you will be eating a "bad" salty meal, what can you do beforehand to help counter this?

_____

_____

_____

_____

_____

_____

_____

_____

_____

_____

_____

"Salt is the second major constituent in our body, next to water. We need adequate amounts of good salt in our diet to run hundreds of different biochemical pathways."

- Dr. David Brownstein

Rotate Your Foods to Get Variety

In order to get proper nutrition, avoid food sensitivities and stay satisfied with your diet; it is important to get a wide variety of foods and rotate your basics often. Eat a variety of colors and add new food regularly.

Eating your favorites often is okay; just mix it up a couple of times each week. For example, in your smoothies, if your favorite greens to use are spinach, use them most of the time but perhaps on the weekends, use kale or Swiss chard. If you love chopped apples in your oatmeal, go ahead, but now and then, use chopped pears instead. Try new fruits and veggies that you haven't used before, both plain and in salads or smoothies. Some foods, like beets, have a very different flavor when cooked than they do raw. Try them roasted. Then try them shredded on a salad. Eat a variety of colors. Try almond or pecan butter instead of peanut butter. Explore a variety of beans, lentils, and grains that can be used on salads, in soups or in wraps.

The most common foods that people are sensitive or allergic to include dairy, corn, soy, wheat, peanuts and sugar.

- What food ruts are you stuck in? What foods do you need to mix up? What could you occasionally use instead? Make a list of at least 3 foods that you have heard about and would like to experiment with, but haven't yet. Circle the one that you will try this week.

Use Medications as a Last Resort

I am not saying that there isn't a place for medication, however, for minor ailments try a few simple natural things first. Many minor symptoms, such as headaches and upset stomachs can be handled quickly and effectively with very little effort.   \

If you need medication, take it but just don't get in the habit of taking Tylenol or Ibuprofen regularly for long periods of time. The next time that you feel a little off (stomach or head ache, sore throat, etc.), try this: drink a full glass of water, find a dark quiet place to lay down, do some deep breathing, and lay perfectly still for at least 20 minutes (longer if possible). If you are at work, just come as close as you can. You may need to take a break and go out to your car. In about 50 percent of cases, this works. Many of our issues are due to stress and dehydration and this remedy addresses both.

You can also keep some peppermint essential oil on hand as this particular oil is one of the most versatile. Essential oils are concentrated plant essences. They have wonderful medicinal properties and work quickly. Peppermint essential oil is great for the relief of minor headaches, sinus issues and stomach discomfort. Just put a drop or two on your temples or on the back of your neck to relieve stress and re-energize?

- What symptoms do you deal with regularly? What could you do ahead of time to <u>prevent</u> these symptoms? For example, if you always have a headache after your Monday afternoon meeting, perhaps Sunday evening and Monday morning you could drink more water, exercise, do some extra deep breathing and come to the meeting more focused and ready to be productive.

_____

_____

_____

_____

_____

_____

_____

_____

_____

_____

"Let food be thy medicine and medicine be thy food."
-Hippocrates

Avoid GMO's

Genetically-modified foods are causing many problems in Americans' health today. They are associated with several inflammatory gut issues, allergies, liver failure, brain fog and fertility/hormone disturbances, to name just a few.

Although there are more and more crops being subject to GMO's all the time the two main GMO crops to avoid are corn and soy. Again, as mentioned before, if you eat mostly whole foods, this will be less of a problem, but if you eat a lot of processed foods, corn and soy are in nearly all of them. Besides being genetically modified, corn is high in sugar and really difficult to digest. Soy is a major hormone disrupter as it increases estrogen, making a person bigger (that's one of the roles of estrogen). Corn may be listed as corn oil, corn syrup, corn flour etc. Soy is often listed as soybean oil, soy lecithin, soy flour etc. It is recommended to avoid corn and soy altogether but if you must partake, be sure to get organic, non-GMO products.

- What are you currently eating that contains corn and soy? List them here. How could you upgrade? For example, instead of corn based tortilla chips, you could use organic rice chips. Next to each corn/soy product, list your healthy alternative.

_____

_____

_____

_____

_____

_____

_____

_____

_____

Eat Less

Most Americans eat about twice the number of calories than the body requires. This causes major fatigue as the body is bogged down and unable to keep up with all of the digesting it needs to do. When we overeat, even on healthy whole foods, the body has to use more of our energy to digest, store, assimilate and eliminate the food. This leaves us with less energy for work, family and fun activities.

You may need to eat fewer snacks, or less dense food, or just smaller quantities at each meal. Use smaller serving dishes and eat slowly. Be conscious of how you feel before you dish up seconds. So often we go back for more for reasons that are social, taste, habit or emotional, rather than actual hunger. If you don't feel hungry, wait for 10 minutes or so. Talk to people, drink water, take some deep breaths. This gives the food that you have already eaten a chance to start digesting and gives you time to evaluate how you really feel. If at that point you still feel hungry, by all means, dish up and savor more food. Just be sure that you are choosing what is best for you at that time.

Keep in mind that organic whole foods give you more nutrition so you need less to be satisfied. This change can take some time to get used to but over time will result in being more satisfied with less food.

- When do you tend to eat too much? At social gatherings? At work? When stressed? On the weekend? When you go out? With certain people? What do you need to do NOW to prepare for these times? How can you think differently about these situations?

_____

_____

_____

_____

_____

_____

_____

_____

_____

_____

_____

"You should get up from the table as light as you sat down to it".
-Gabriel Cousens

Section 3 – Habits That You Put in Your Life

The habits that you put in your LIFE will increase your energy, productivity, and create a more amazing YOU. Your lifestyle is made up of habits, either positive or negative that allow you to be able to make quick decisions easily. People who have a lifestyle made up of positive habits are more efficient, have more energy and overall get more out of life! Choose one to start TODAY!

Sleep

Getting enough sleep and enough good quality sleep is a game changer when it comes to having vitality and being productive.

There are several things that are important to keep in mind in regard to great, restful sleep. First, your body does its best healing between 10 p.m. and 6 a.m. while you sleep, therefore it is ideal to be in bed by 10 p.m. whenever possible.

If you aren't sleeping, you aren't getting the optimal healing and repairing that your body needs on a regular basis. Think of it like cleaning your house. You don't clean the gutters every day; that would be more of an annual or semiannual task. But what would happen if you stopped doing your laundry or cleaning your dirty dishes or some other daily task? After a while, you would have a bigger problem on your hands. If you don't get that healing and repair, eventually your body will be overloaded with toxins and you will feel sick.

Several reasons that make sleep difficult include eating before bed, not winding down, exercising before bed, going to bed stressed, watching TV (especially intense or violent images-this can include the news), noise in the sleeping area and too much sugar during the day. A few things that help you sleep well include exercising in the morning, a healthy, whole food diet, lavender essential oil, soft music, chamomile tea, a good wind down routine and a hot bath or shower. When you have a lot to do, in most cases, it is better to go to bed early and get up earlier than to stay up late.

- Describe your current sleep habits. What could you do to improve them? Get an action plan here. Be specific. For example, if you are currently going to bed at mid-night, what would have to happen for you to be in bed by 11 PM? Start with the easiest steps first to build momentum.

_____

_____

_____

_____

_____

_____

_____

_____

_____

_____

Quiet Time and Meditation

Blocking out a few minutes each day for quiet time, meditation or prayer, reading scripture, visualizing your ideal life or thinking on a few quotes or verses while taking long deep breaths can be a helpful tool for maintaining balance in your overall life, leaving you less stressed and more fully present wherever you are. Although this is a great habit to do in the morning, do it wherever and whenever it fits for you. It may be something that you do in your car on a lunch break or before you go to bed at night. This should not feel like work. Instead, it should be a re-charge for your body, mind and spirit. Think of it as a daily mini-retreat.

- Routine is key. Choose a place and time you know you will be able to consistently have quiet for at least a few moments. Decide what you will do and if you will need anything (Bible, journal, music, cushion to sit on, etc.). Get it set up. Now, choose at least one positive statement or verse that you can focus on and record it here.

_____

_____

_____

_____

_____

_____

_____

_____

_____

_____

_____

Don't Stay Stuck; Build a Team!

We were not designed to do everything on our own. Know your limitations and know when you need to ask for help. Start building a team of trusted individuals who you can count on when you need help or advice. Your team may include a business consultant, financial advisor, pastor, teacher, holistic doctor and dentist, massage therapist, nutritionist, baby sitter, and some great friends. No matter where you are feeling stuck, just don't stay stuck long. If you aren't feeling well, or just need a break, call on the appropriate "team member" to help you move forward.

- Who do you already have on your team of trusted advisors/helpers? Who do you need to add? List them here.

_____

_____

_____

_____

_____

_____

_____

_____

_____

_____

_____

_____

"No man is an island"

-John Donne

Party Time!

Plan time for fun. This could be something as elaborate as taking a 7 night cruise or more simple things like a date night with your spouse. Or it could be having friends over or sharing a "funny story of the week" every Monday morning at the office.

You may be wondering what this has to do with increasing your efficiency. Laughter is an incredible stress reducer. It clears the mind and allows you to return to your daily life fresher and with more energy and creativity. If you have ever been to see a really good comedian, you know what I mean. No matter how anxious or stressed you are when you go in, after laughing hysterically for a solid hour, you leave feeling like you just had a mini-vacation.

For some this will be an easy one and will come naturally. For others, it will be something that you will need to be intentional about or it won't happen. Don't worry, with a little practice you will find yourself laughing freely in no time!

- Create a list of at least 10 things that you have fun doing (or think you would have fun doing). Include some big things (vacations), some "medium" things (overnight at a local bed and breakfast) and some daily things (going to a comedy show, getting together with fun friends or trying something new). Then, get out your calendar and put at least one "party" on the schedule in the next 10 days, another in the next 30 days and one in the next 6 months.

_____

_____

_____

_____

_____

_____

_____

_____

_____

_____

"Against the assault of laughter nothing can stand."
-Mark Twain

Get a Grip on Stress and Anxiety

Stress and anxiety are amongst the top reasons that Americans visit their doctors each year. There are however many natural actions that you can take to reduce stress and anxiety. Let's start with stress that we bring upon ourselves. This would be, for example, feeling overwhelmed because you are always late. Of course, there are lots of practical steps that you can take to eliminate this stress, such as setting your clocks 5-10 minutes earlier than the actual time, do more at night to prepare for the next day, leave extra travel time and set your alarm 15 minutes earlier. If you actually do these things, the worst thing that would happen is that you would get to work early and have a few moments to sip tea or get things done so you feel ahead of the game when everyone else shows up!

There is also stress that you don't have control over such as a traffic jam or a power outage. For these situations, it is best to have a plan for what you will do when these things come up. Some examples could include deep breathing, reminding yourself that you are only responsible for what you can control and finding the good in the challenge (something you are learning, a new perspective, or things to be grateful for). One additional aspect that is really important is supporting the body nutritionally so that it can stand up under unusual occasional stresses. The body was not created to stay up working late every night. However, on occasion (end of year audits for example), this should be no problem if you have prepared your body adequately.

In general, regular exercise, proper nutrition, adequate amounts of pure water and deep breathing are key. Keeping up with these things daily is like putting a few dollars into your bank account each day. Then, when an unexpected bill comes up, you have enough to pay it without going into debt. Think of your nutrition this way. But what if you are in major stress right now and you aren't prepared? Is there anything you can do? Yes, of course, you will just need more of those basics. Start now and don't stop until about 5 days after you feel back to normal. When you are under stress, regardless of whether it is mental (writing a presentation), physical (staying up late to work on a deadline) or emotional (worried about a loved one), you use up your nutrients much quicker than usual. This means that to keep up, you will need more nutrition. Notice that you don't need more food, just more nutrition. This is where some healthy fats and greens powder (or green smoothies) can be especially helpful. Digestion shuts down when you are under lots of stress so it is important to eat light, easy to digest foods during these times.

- Where do you see that you are creating stress? What specific steps can you take to change this? What areas of your life are you struggling to respond well to (emotional, physical, mental, etc.) stress in? How can you support your body with basic nutrition during this time?

_____

_____

_____

_____

_____

_____

_____

_____

_____

_____

_____

Deep Breathing

Deep breathing is an amazing equalizer and stress buster. It tends to have an adaptogenic effect on the body. In other words, if you're feeling anxious, it will calm you down and relax you. If you're feeling tired and sluggish, it will tend to perk you up. When you control your breathing, you tend to have better control over your emotions as well. Ideally, when possible, do some deep breathing outside in fresh air. Here is a simple deep breathing exercise: breathe in for four counts, hold your breath for four counts, then exhale slowly for four counts. Repeat this at least four times. Repeat several times throughout the day for optimal benefits.

• Where, in your day, do you most need to do this exercise? How will you remember to do this? Place reminders where you need them (in your car, kitchen, at your desk, etc). Also, start <u>and</u> end your day with a few deep breaths.

_____

_____

_____

_____

_____

_____

_____

_____

_____

_____

_____

"Deep breathing signals your brain that you're going to be okay which helps every function in the body work more efficiently"
- LeAnn Fritz

Relationships

Relationships can be a source of great pain and frustration, or profound joy and satisfaction. In order for a relationship to be positive it will take effort over time. This looks different with your coworkers, than with your spouse, parents, children or neighbor. Each individual relationship will require different types of investments. Strained relationships, regardless of who they are with, as you have probably experienced, can affect all areas of one's life. If you are struggling with your marriage, you tend to be out of focus and not present at work. Likewise, if you have trouble with an employer or co-worker, it can be challenging not to bring that home. This constant stress on your mind leaves you struggling to focus and be effective no matter where you are.

To eliminate this, invest in people, own your part of any issues, and move forward quickly so your life is changed for the better, rather than bogged down by the constant nagging in your mind about what you should have said or what the person said to you. These are not powerful and productive thoughts. Relationships are most successful when all the people involved are thinking about, encouraging and serving each other, rather than merely looking out for their own interests.

- Do a brief evaluation of the relationships in your life with friends, family members, and coworkers. Are any of them strained? If so, how have you contributed? What are 3 steps you can take to make things better with that person? If you currently don't have any strained relationships, what can you do in general to invest in those people who you most love and respect? Send a note of appreciation? Give a gift? Invite them to dinner?

Have a Morning Routine

Starting your day right can have dramatic results on the quality and quantity of things you accomplish the rest of the day. Getting in the habit of nourishing yourself before you even leave the house in the morning will give you the fuel you need to serve others throughout the day, both at work and at home. You can decide what is most important and what you want to prioritize into your morning.

If you are a morning person, get up early and pack a lot in. If you are not, just keep it simple and start out by giving yourself just three simple habits in the morning. Here is a short list of some options for your morning routine: drink 32 oz. of lemon water, make a green smoothie (or other healthy breakfast), take supplements, read, exercise, deep breathing, make a list for the day, drink tea, pack a healthy lunch, meditation/prayer/scripture reading, visualize and write in a journal.

- Are you a morning person? If not, choose three simple things that you could do each morning to enrich your day. If yes, choose 4-8 things that you could add. Keep in mind that many of these take very little time (drink water, take supplements, etc.). Record your action steps here, then post them elsewhere so you will be reminded each morning.

_____

_____

_____

_____

_____

_____

_____

_____

_____

_____

_____

If you start right, by feeding your mind, body and spirit, you will have greater energy, be more focused and get more done the rest of your day.

- LeAnn Fritz

Have an Evening Routine

Evening is a time to prepare for tomorrow and reflect on today. Depending on your schedule and preferences, there are many ways to do this. There are three parts to the evening routine: reflecting on the current day, preparing for tomorrow, and unwinding for a great night of sleep. If you're a night person, spend more time in the evening routine and get a lot in. If you're not, keep it simple and just add a few steps to your evening.

Reflecting on the day is a great way to evaluate and see if you are happy with your accomplishments, or if you may need to make adjustments for tomorrow. You can do this by journaling, talking to a friend or spouse, or just by going for a walk and thinking about it. Just remember that the goal is not to beat yourself up if you're not happy with the outcomes for the day. The goal is to learn for the sake of taking new actions the next day.

Next is preparing for the next day. This could include: cleaning up the kitchen, packing your lunch for tomorrow, making a list, picking out clothes, doing laundry, gathering things that you will need to bring with you the next day and setting them by the door so you don't forget them, loading the car, etc. On some days, this may take a while but for the most part, it can be a quick but helpful addition to your routine.

The final part of the evening routine is the unwinding. This doesn't have to be a massage and a 2 hour bath (although that may be delightful). It can be as simple as sitting on the porch with a cup of tea, cuddling with your spouse while you talk about the day, listening to relaxing music while you do some deep breathing, or journaling about your goals and victories. It is important to do this even if you can only fit in a few minutes for it. The purpose of all of this is to relax and settle in for the day in a way that allows you to sleep well and wake up prepared and organized for the next day.

- Let's create your evening routine. List two actions that you can take to reflect on your day. List two actions that you can take to prepare for the next day. List two actions that you can take to relax and unwind so you can sleep well and wake up feeling great.

_____

_____

_____

_____

_____

_____

_____

_____

_____

_____

_____

"Tomorrow starts tonight. Prepare tonight for a powerful tomorrow."
-LeAnn Fritz

Eating Habits

When possible, eat as close as you can to the same time each day. Seek to have a 12-hour fast each night. For example, if you finish dinner at 6 PM, don't eat until at least 6 AM the next morning. This gives the body time to clean, heal, repair and digest yesterday's food before you start eating for today.

Seek not to eat late at night. Eat little-to-nothing for at least 2-3 hours before you go to bed. Before each meal, pause and take three long deep slow breaths before your first bite. Chew slowly and thoroughly. Eat in a quiet place where you can focus on your food rather than in your car or at your desk. These actions allow you to de-stress a bit before you eat so your food can be better digested. If you are under lots of stress, green juices or smoothies are best since your digestion won't be at its highest peak. They give you lots of nutrition but are "pre-digested" so your body won't have to work as hard to break them down. Drink lots of water between meals, but very little with meals, so that your stomach acid isn't diluted. Eating this way allows for optimal digestion and assimilation which yields better focus and concentration.

- Choose three of the healthy eating habits listed here that would help you the most. List them here. Is there anything specific you need to do to accomplish this? Record that here as well (such as blocking out time for lunch so no meetings get scheduled).

_____

_____

_____

_____

_____

_____

_____

_____

_____

_____

_____

Be Prepared

When you are seeking to live a healthy lifestyle for optimal energy and efficiency, it is important to be prepared. Have water and some healthy snacks in your car, in your office and easy to grab at home. This way if you are stuck at work later than expected, or in your car caught in a traffic jam, you never have to go hungry or cave in and eat poor quality foods. Trail mixes made from dried fruit and raw nuts and seeds are great to have on hand. Fresh, easy to grab fruit is great too (apples, pears, bananas).

If you know that you will be going to a lunch or dinner meeting or a social gathering where there won't be many healthy options, eat before you go. Even if you just have a snack, you will be less likely to eat junk food, and even if you do, you will likely consume less than if you walk in hungry. Drink a large bottle or glass of water before you go as well so you are well hydrated. If it's appropriate, you could also bring a healthy whole food dish to pass as well. This could be something as simple as a cut up watermelon or something more time consuming like homemade spicy beans and rice.

Although food and nutrition is one important factor, we should also have strategies in mind that prepare us for handling perceived failures. Stress from a traffic jam, getting to the gym and having no motivation to work out and even positive stresses like getting a promotion or finding out you're being re-located to your favorite city in the U.S. can all bump us off our good schedule if we aren't prepared. This is why it is important to view your life holistically and nourish all areas of your life so that you are preemptively ready for any challenge. The idea here isn't to eliminate all trials forever. You will always have challenges, however, those challenges will be easier to handle as you develop more balance and have more tools in your arsenal to handle what life brings.

- Where do you need to keep a stash of healthy snacks? What will you put there? Are there any consistent pitfalls that you can identify so you can do some preventative work? If so, list them here, along with some possible solutions.

_____

_____

_____

_____

_____

_____

_____

_____

_____

_____

_____

"You will always have challenges, however, those challenges will be easier to handle as you develop more balance and have more tools in your arsenal to handle what life brings."

-LeAnn Fritz

Exercise vs. Physical Activity

After earning an undergraduate degree in Exercise Science and spending seven years as a certified personal trainer, there is one thing that is very clear to me. Physical activity and exercise are both important but they are not the same.

Physical activity includes gardening, house work, getting the mail, cleaning the garage and playing with children. These activities get the body moving but do not serve as regular exercise. Exercise works the cardiovascular system or the muscular system for an extended period of time. This includes: brisk walking, running, biking, dancing, swimming, weight lifting and aerobics. Exercise is magical. It reduces stress, burns calories, increases digestion and proper elimination, tones the body, strengthens the heart, improves mood, lymphatic flow, promotes healthy elimination and so much more. If you are currently exercising, keep it up! Add variety in either intensity or type of exercise. For example, if you love to walk, occasionally change the intensity (walk up hills or jog) or the type of exercise (bike or swim). Be sure to get some weight lifting in too. A muscle responds best if you vary the type of stress you put on it, a concept called muscle confusion. This is why you often get results when you first start exercising but then if you continue doing the same thing, the results taper off a bit.

If you're not exercising at all, start with something sustainable, like 10 minutes of walking four days per week and build up from there. The primary goal here is to build the habit. In my years as a personal trainer, many people would consider their physical activity as exercise and often feel like their progress was coming slower than once they started doing both!

• Describe your current exercise habits. What is the next step for you? Do you need to exercise more often? Add intensity? Do something different? Do you prefer to exercise alone? With music? With a friend? What do you need to do to get started? If you are not exercising now, when will you start?

_____

_____

_____

_____

_____

_____

_____

_____

_____

_____

Journal

Journaling can be a great way to keep track of things you want to do, including your goals and aspirations. You can use your journal however you like. It can be a success journal where you record quotes and tips about reaching your goals or a victory journal where you record areas you had victory each day. You can use it as a gratitude journal, which can be very helpful when you are feeling stressed or depressed. You could use it as a diary to just get your thoughts and feelings out. Or, you could use it as any combination of these ideas.

• What type of journaling do you prefer? Typing on the computer, note
  book, picture journal (great for artistic people)? When is a good time
  for you to journal? Weekends, evenings, mornings? What do you think
  would be most helpful for you to record?

_____

_____

_____

_____

_____

_____

_____

_____

_____

_____

_____

*"Don't use your mind for a filing cabinet. Use your mind to work out
problems and find answers; file away good ideas in your journal."*
                                                    - Jim Rohn

Finances/Budget

If you don't think that your personal finances play a huge role in all areas of life, let me ask you this: have you ever received a bill that you literally didn't have the money to pay? Or have you ever had a loved one with a legitimate need that you wanted desperately to help them with, but couldn't? It is a terrible feeling that sticks with you throughout the day. You think about it often and it can be hard to focus on what you are doing at work, home or wherever you are.

Perhaps you have no trouble paying your bills, but want to move into a freedom stage with your finances. More money yields more freedom. In this stage, you can save for your dream house, car, give to organizations, or to church functions or family members who are in need. You are free both financially but also mentally free from having to worry or think about how you will get by.

Regardless of where you are on your financial path, you will need a plan to get to the next step. You want to be fully aware of your financial goals and plans, giving every dollar a destination rather than just spending randomly and hoping you get where you want to be. Having a financial plan helps to clear your mind. You don't have to worry. You just need to work the plan. A clear mind is more productive in every facet of life.

- How would you describe your current financial picture? What do you need to do to get to the next level? Do you need to sell something? Seek the help of a financial planner? What is one thing you could do to save money now? Shop your car insurance? Buy gifts when they are on sale? Plan ahead when booking travel to save money? What is one thing that you could do to make more money now?

_____

_____

_____

_____

_____

_____

_____

_____

_____

_____

Serve Others

Who can you serve? Serving and helping others is an incredible habit to add to your life. Serving others can open doors for you. It makes you feel great. It is a great antidote to feeling depressed about your own circumstances. This can take many forms ranging from volunteering at your local school or homeless shelter to mowing your neighbors lawn to taking time to talk to a friend who is going through a tough time. Everyone wins when you seek to serve. Serving others is more than just an action, it's an attitude and way of thinking. Always be asking, "How and who can I help?"

- Who can you serve? Who in your life has a need that you could help with? (A coworker? Family member? Neighbor? Someone at school? Church?) If you don't know of anyone personally, what local causes do you believe in that you could help with? (Homeless shelter, blood drives, tutoring children, etc.).

_____

_____

_____

_____

_____

_____

_____

_____

_____

_____

Clutter Busting Schedule

For work and home (and even your car if you need to) each week, include de-cluttering in your schedule. If you haven't already noticed from the work you have been doing in the action steps, routine is an important component of getting things done in a productive and efficient way.

Part of your routine will include de-cluttering your space. Just like in your home, you may do dishes daily, laundry weekly and only clean the gutters once a year. The same holds true for all of your spaces. At your office, choose a time each day to just put away basics. This should take 5 minutes or less, ideally at the end of your workday. This way, you are starting each day fresh.

Once each week, preferably at the end of the week, block out 20-30 minutes to clean your desk, tie up loose ends and clear any clutter that has accumulated. Do this same thing for your house, car and any other space where you are regularly spending time. Here is the key though, you have to schedule this; set a reminder, a timer then DO IT. Otherwise, it's just a nice idea that won't actually make you more energized and productive.

• List the physical areas of your life that need some clutter control. For each one, plan the best way to do this. In most cases, it's a few minutes each day, 20-60 minutes each week and perhaps a half or full day a couple of times per year. Schedule this in. Write a powerful, positive statement about how this will help you succeed.

_____

_____

_____

_____

_____

_____

_____

_____

_____

_____

_____

_____

"There is an inextricable link between mental and physical clutter,"
-Virginia Barkely

Get Outside

There are several benefits to being outside. First, you have the fresh air. Outdoor air is almost always cleaner than indoor air. Taking a few deep breaths outside can clear your lungs as well as calm your mind. Next, the sunshine gives a healthy dose of vitamin D. Spend 30-60 minutes in the sun any day that you can if you live in a climate that allows for it. The more of your skin that's exposed the better so if you can, get on your swim suit and head for the beach (or just the back yard). Vitamin D elevates the mood, decreases depression and gives a major boost to the immune system. For one hour or less, you don't need to be concerned about sunscreen. The vitamin D will not usually penetrate it. Finally, having your bare feet in the grass or sand (also known as grounding) is helpful for decreasing inflammation and improving mental clarity. If you can't get outside for a long period of time, maybe you could just walk outside for 5 minutes on a lunch break or eat your lunch outside at a local park.

*   How do you like to spend your time outside? At the beach? In the woods? Exercising? List 3 ways that you could sneak more outside time into your schedule. Circle the one that you will apply first.

_____

_____

_____

_____

_____

_____

_____

_____

_____

_____

"Keep your face to the sunshine and you cannot see a shadow,"
-Helen Keller

Cravings

Where do cravings come from? Cravings are not random. They can stem from emotional or physical roots. They are the mind or body's way of asking for something you are lacking. In the case of emotional cravings, you may tend to crave sweets during difficult times when your life is lacking sweetness. The craving for higher fat foods on the other hand is usually associated with the desire for insulation or protection from something. With cravings that are more physical there is usually a nutrient that is depleted. For example, when you crave chocolate, your body probably needs magnesium. Most people are low in magnesium and chocolate has lots of it. It would be ideal to eat raw organic cacao nibs because most chocolate is so processed and full of sugar that you get way more than just magnesium. However, if that is all your body knows that has high magnesium, that is what it will crave. When you crave salty foods, like chips, cheese, crackers and processed meats you are probably lacking natural sodium. Instead, eat more celery and dark leafy greens such as spinach, kale and chard. The craving will usually go away rather quickly. If it doesn't, it is highly likely that the craving is indeed emotional in nature. The reason this is important to know is that if you have an understanding of the real need, you will know the REAL way to satisfy it with REAL food. Then, you feel nourished and the craving goes away.

- What foods do you find yourself craving? List them here. Next to each one record if you believe it to be primarily an emotional or nutritional issue. Then record what you can do to alleviate it in the most nutritious way.

_____

_____

_____

_____

_____

_____

_____

_____

_____

_____

Time for Detox and Rejuvenation

Plan time as often as possible, but at least one-two times per year, to go away for detoxification and restoration. A couple of years ago, I went to a healing center for a detox retreat and was able to restore and re-balance after a time of high stress. Although you can do this at home to some degree, it is far safer and more effective to do this under the care of a holistic practitioner and also away from the regular stresses of life. This will be a time of resting and clearing the mind so you can come back stronger and more effective in your family, career and overall life. You can do these retreats on your own or with a group of friends. Just be sure that whomever you invite will be positive and uplifting to you. At these retreats you may learn a variety of skill such as: how to eat well, breath properly, make amazing food, juice fast, and much more, depending on where you go. If you can't take a full week, go for a long weekend. This will sharpen the mind, body and spirit and you will come back feeling light, clear minded, and energized, to accomplish more than ever before.

Get Healthy NOW Action Steps

* When was the last time that you did some detoxification? Record how long you would like to go (2 days, 4 days, 7 days) and when would work best for you. What would be your primary goal for this time? (Weight loss, stress reduction, rest, increasing energy etc)

_____

_____

_____

_____

_____

_____

_____

_____

_____

_____

_____

Make a New Habit Checklist

When you are working to be the best YOU that you can be, there is often a feeling of overwhelm when you consider all of the wonderful new things that you want to put into your mind, body and lifestyle. Where do you start and how do you remember it all? Don't worry. After a few weeks, many of these new behaviors will become habits and you won't even have to think about them.

Here is a great way to get started: on a blank sheet of paper, or a spreadsheet if you'd rather use a computer, create a checklist. On the left side, list your new goals, behaviors and habits. Along the top, list the dates for the next 30 days. Then, each day, keep your list nearby and check things off as you complete them. This will help you keep track of your victories and will give you a sense of accomplishment at the end of the day when you see all of the great things that you are doing.

Get Healthy NOW Action Steps

- Make your list of new habits you plan to add. Start with the most important or easiest ones for you, and don't worry about doing everything in the first few weeks. Also, if there is something that you are already doing, don't add it. Now, use that list to create your chart. Make notes of how amazing you feel with each passing day!

_____

_____

_____

_____

_____

_____

_____

_____

_____

_____

Conclusion

Congratulations! You have just nourished your mind, body and life by learning 60 ways to fuel your energy, increase your productivity and improve your overall life. You have gained an understanding of what you need to add to your body, mind and lifestyle to reach your potential. You are already, in part, transformed! If you follow the habits and changes recommended in this book, every area of your life will benefit. But with so much information, how do you process it? What is the best way to start? The best way is to choose one step at a time and make it a habit before you move on.

- List one step that you will take to fuel your mind. List one step that you will add to fuel your body. List one habit that you will add to your life for becoming the most optimal version of yourself.

_____

_____

_____

_____

_____

_____

_____

_____

_____

_____

_____

"A journey of a thousand miles begins with a single step."
-Lao-tzu

Note From LeAnn:

Dear Reader,
Again, congratulations for taking the time to read this book. I am so excited for the transformations that will be taking place in your life. I would love to hear about them. Please send me a note about the great changes that you have made to: info@newhopehealth.net and add MY STORY in the subject line.

Resources:
Vitamix Blender:
Vitamix Blenders are the GOLD STANDARD for blenders in the health food industry. You can make so many delicious and healthy meals with this wonderful machine. As an affiliate, you can use my special code to receive free shipping off any Vitamix Blender that you choose. You can use it on the web site www.vitamix.com or by calling direct at 1-800-848-2649. Either way, use this code 06-005027 (to save $25 on shipping)! You won't regret this incredible health investment.

Supplements:
Due to the great deal of confusion around natural health supplements, I wanted to offer some help so that you can get the greatest benefit from the supplements you take without having to worry if you are taking something harmful or ineffective. I have done extensive research and use only the purest, cleanest and most effective herbs and supplements for myself and my clients. I have gathered these supplements in one place and made them available through an on-line store to make it more convenient for those who are ready to take their health to the next level.

Because there is not adequate space in this book to go into detail about this, I have created a free download for you about supplements that will help you in three ways. First, it will tell you what to look for and avoid in any supplements that you take. Second, it will give you an overview of the top 10 supplements that I personally use and recommend for most people. Finally, you will also receive a coupon for 10% off your first purchase. To get these great gifts, go to www.NewHopeHealth.com

Appendix A

Superfood list: This is a brief list of some of the more common superfoods and just a few of their benefits. There are many more superfoods that you can enjoy.

*There are also lots of superfood mixes and powders that combine several superfoods into one product that you can add to smoothies or other foods or drinks.

Information on GMO's (Genetically Modified Organisms):
Jeffrey Smith's web site http://responsibletechnology.org

Superfood	Good For
Goji berries	Energy, longevity, alkalinizing, brain fuel
Spirilina	Protein, minerals and detoxification
Chlorella	Protein, minerals and detoxification, especially heavy metals
Maca	Energy, libido and hormone balancing
Hemp seeds	Healthy fats, protein
Chia seeds	Healthy fats, protein and calcium
Bee Pollen	Energy, protein, minerals, allergies and hormone balancing
Medicinal mushrooms (coryceps, reishi etc)	Energy, immunity and overall longevity